VICTORIA NATURA

Medicinal Mushrooms

Unlocking The Power of Nature's Medicine

First edition

This book was professionally typeset on Reedsy.
Find out more at reedsy.com

Contents

1

The Purpose of this Book for the Reader

This book aims to educate and inform readers about the incredible health benefits of medicinal mushrooms and how to choose a high-quality supplement. Throughout the pages of this book, you will learn about the history and traditional use of medicinal mushrooms, as well as the various types of mushrooms and their unique health benefits. You will discover the science behind the active compounds in these fascinating fungi and how they can support overall health and wellness. This book will provide you with the knowledge and tools you need to make an informed decision when choosing a medicinal mushroom supplement, including what to look for in terms of quality and potency. By the end of this book, you will have a deeper understanding of the power of medicinal mushrooms and how they can enhance your health and well-being.

2

A Brief History of Medicinal Mushrooms

Although often overlooked or generally unknown, mushrooms have long been utilized therapeutically across many civilizations. Mushrooms were sought after and used to treat anything, from minor ailments like the common cold to more serious ones like cancer.

The first reported usage of mushrooms for medical purposes dates back to the Egyptians around 1550 BCE. Mushrooms were also used for their medicinal advantages by the ancient Greeks and Romans, who suggested using them to treat diseases and wounds. One of the essential herbal texts of its time, De Materia Medica, by the legendary herbalist Dioscorides, even had a recipe for a "mushroom ointment."

While in Asia, mushrooms have long been employed in traditional Chinese medicine (TCM) to keep the body balanced and ward off disease. Each organ has a relationship with a season and an emotion, according to TCM theory. The liver and kidney, related to the autumn and the water element, are nourished by mushrooms. They are said to aid in calming down unpleasant feelings like resentment and rage.

Many medicinal mushrooms contain antioxidants and polysaccharides (a carbohydrate that provides numerous health benefits), which help boost immunity and protect cells from damage. They're also a natural source of umami—a savory flavor that can make food more satisfying—which can help reduce cravings and promote weight loss. Additionally, some studies have shown that certain mushrooms may help lower cholesterol levels, manage diabetes, protect against specific types of cancer (such as breast cancer), and improve cognitive function.

While all mushroom species boast health benefits, some are more potent than others regarding medicinal use. Common varieties like white button mushrooms don't pack as much of a punch nutritionally as more unusual types like Chaga or shiitake mushrooms. However, they can still be part of a healthy diet. When it comes to medicinal use, however, you'll want to focus on species like reishi, cordyceps, maitake, lion's mane, and turkey tails—all of which have historically treated various ailments.

Despite frequently being disregarded in favor of more well-known herbs like echinacea or ginger root, societies worldwide have utilized mushrooms as medicine for ages due to their health-improving qualities. Supplementing medicinal mush-rooms is an effective option to prevent sickness or mediate symptoms while sick.

Health Benefits Of Medicinal Mushrooms Overview

This chapter provides an excellent overview of some of the most popular medicinal mushrooms. Mushrooms are known for their delicious taste, commonly experienced throughout the world. The health benefits of medicinal mushrooms are potent and beneficial for people's daily lives.

The anti-inflammatory effect of mushrooms significantly improves the immune system's efficiency. Mushrooms help stimulate macrophages in your immune system, which enhances its ability to defeat foreign bodies and make you less prone to severe illnesses.

Mushrooms contain a significant amount of potassium, the nutrient that reduces sodium's negative impact on your body. Potassium can also lessen tension in your blood vessels, which helps in lowering blood pressure.

Mushrooms complement chemotherapy and radiation therapy by countering side effects of cancer, like nausea, anemia, bone marrow suppression, and lowered resistance. For these reasons, chemo patients consume mushrooms to help alleviate unfortunate side effects.

Mushrooms have therapeutic properties that help lower cholesterol, especially in overweight adults. Also, they contain compounds and nutrients that prevent the cells from sticking to the blood vessel walls, often leading to plaque build-up. These health benefits help the heart maintain healthy blood circulation and blood pressure.

Lion's Mane and reishi, tested through scientific trials, demonstrate the importance of using medicinal mushrooms for managing neurodegenerative diseases like Alzheimer's.

Not only can mushrooms protect the brain from neurodegeneration, but they can also boost cognitive function, improve focus and memory and even boost mood. Mushrooms, like Cordyceps, lion's Mane, and reishi, have adaptogenic properties that can reduce the adverse effects of stress on the body.

Compounds in mushrooms, especially beta-glucan, act as prebiotics, all of which fuel the growth of healthy gut bacteria and promote a favorable gut environment. A healthy gut plays a crucial role in maintaining your immune defenses, digesting food, and communicating with your brain through hormones and nerves.

Chaga mushroom is an adaptogen that helps the body adapt to occasional stress. Often used for supporting the immune system, skin, and healthy digestion, as well as natural cleansing processes of the body.

Cordyceps is an adaptogen that supports a healthy response to the occasional stress. It also supports energy and stamina, sexual health, kidney health, and lung health. Many athletes have begun to supplement cordyceps mushrooms and touted its benefits of drastically improving their athletic performance.

Lion's Mane supplements support memory and cognitive function. It also offers nourishment for your brain and supports nerve growth factor production. There health compounds in Lions Mane mushrooms, known as hericenones and erinacines, are attributed to their brain-boosting benefits.

Maitake Mushroom

Maitake, also known as hen of the woods mushroom, is used to support nervous system health, cardiovascular health, immune health, and healthy digestive function. Scientific studies have revealed the benefits of maitake supporting healthy blood sugar levels and liver health.

Poria mushroom promotes a healthy immune function, the body's natural transition to a healthy night's sleep, normal hydration levels, relaxation, memory, normal stomach function, and nervous system health. This mushroom's medicinal dates back as a health elixir used by Native Americans.

Reishi is an adaptogenic mushroom that supports longevity. It helps with the body's occasional stress response, cardiovascular, immune, and nervous systems, kidney and liver health, relaxation, and healthy sleep. People have touted the Reishi mushroom for its ability to regulate their moods.

This mushroom is known for its nutrition and contains vitamins D and B. This mushroom can support cardiovascular, liver, and immune health.

Turkey Tail, which often grows on deciduous trees, supports the immune system, liver health, and gut. Taoists had an exceptionally high opinion of this mushroom because they believed it absorbed the "yang" energy of the roots of the trees.

4

Adaptogens: Powerful Supplements for Reducing Stress

Adaptogens are medicinal herbs that help the body cope with stress by enhancing the body's physiological reaction, and the wide-ranging impacts stress has on physical, emotional, and mental well-being. While under pressure, they may help restore stability to the body's energy levels, hormone levels, and other processes, which can become affected. Adaptogens are popular herbs used in Chinese and Ayurvedic medicine for decades to help the body cope with stress and create increased energy and stamina.

Adaptogen is a term that means "to adjust." It's a term that refers to a group of substances thought to lower the body's stress reaction to tiredness and boost energy and endurance. Adaptogens don't target a hormone or neurotransmitter; they balance activity across the body, resulting in a soothing effect. This enables a person to adapt and manage physical and mental pressures.

Adaptogen is commonly used to describe some of the mushrooms' more potent health advantages. Numerous mushroom species, including lion's mane and cordyceps, may be called adaptogens. The term "adaptogenic" refers to these mushrooms since they can benefit one's neural system, hormone levels, and immune system. Certain types of cancer are also supported with the help of these varieties.

Types of Adaptogens

Turkey Tail is a potent medicinal fungus that incorporates the virtues of many other mushrooms. It is traditionally used to enhance the immune system. Turkey Tail is high in antioxidants, which help combat and prevent cellular damage, and prebiotics, which help with digestion.

Lion's mane has treated many disorders, including dementia and cognitive function. A clinical investigation showed Lion's Mane to have anti-depressant, anti-anxiety, and anti-fatigue properties in older adults with moderate cognitive impairment. Furthermore, the research found that people who received a lion's mane improved their cognitive performance.

Shiitake mushrooms are not only an excellent ingredient in many dishes, but they also provide several health advantages. Several studies have shown Shiitake mushrooms to be good for heart and liver health, immune function, and blood sugar levels, among other things. Studies have proven to reverse the age-related loss in immunological function effectively. They are low in fat, cholesterol, and calories and are high in fiber and B-complex vitamins.

Cordyceps is a powerful adaptogenic fungus that has been around for centuries. It helps to increase energy and endurance. As a result of their ability to make more adenosine triphosphate, these mushrooms make cells more active and help them take in more oxygen. Cordyceps also has immune-boosting properties, assisting your body in fighting off infections and germs.

5

Lions Mane Mushroom Medicinal Properties and Health Benefits

Lion's Mane Mushroom (Hericium Erinaceus) is an edible fungus used for medicinal purposes for centuries in traditional Chinese and Japanese medicine. In recent years, scientific research has shown that Lion's Mane Mushroom contains various compounds with therapeutic properties, making it a promising natural remedy for different health conditions. In this chapter, we will explore the medicinal properties of Lion's Mane Mushrooms and the scientific evidence behind them.

Brain Health and Cognitive Function

One of the most significant health benefits of Lion's Mane Mushroom is its positive impact on brain health and cognitive function. Studies have shown that compounds in this mushroom, such as hericystin and erinacine, have neuroprotective properties that can help improve memory, concentration, and overall brain function.

In one study, mice fed a diet supplemented with Lion's Mane Mushroom extract showed improved cognitive function and increased nerve growth factor (NGF) production. This protein is essential for the growth and survival of neurons. Another human study found that consuming Lion's Mane Mushroom extract daily for 16 weeks significantly improved mild cognitive impairment. This condition often precedes the development of dementia and Alzheimer's disease.

Anti-inflammatory Properties

Lion's Mane Mushroom is also known for its anti-inflammatory properties, which can be beneficial in reducing the risk of various chronic diseases such as heart disease, cancer, and diabetes. The compounds present in this mushroom, such as polysaccharides, beta-glucans, and ergosterols, have been shown to have anti-inflammatory effects by reducing the production of pro-inflammatory cytokines and enzymes.

In a study conducted on mice, Lion's Mane Mushroom extract was found to have a significant anti-inflammatory effect, reducing the production of cytokines and enzymes responsible for inflammation. Another study found that the polysaccharides present in this mushroom could reduce inflammation in human cells and improve the function of immune cells, suggesting a potential role for Lion's Mane Mushroom in boosting the immune system.

Cardiovascular Health

Lion's Mane Mushroom may also positively impact cardio-vascular health by reducing the risk of heart disease. This mushroom contains compounds such as beta-glucans and eritadenine, which have been shown to have cholesterol-lowering properties and improve blood circulation.

A study in rats found that supplementing the diet with Lion's Mane Mushroom extract significantly reduced blood cholesterol levels and improved blood circulation. Another human study found that consuming Lion's Mane Mushroom extract daily for four weeks decreased systolic blood pressure, indicating a potential role for this mushroom in reducing the risk of heart disease.

Antioxidant Properties

Lion's Mane Mushroom is also rich in antioxidants, compounds that protect the body against damage caused by harmful molecules called free radicals. Antioxidants can help reduce the risk of chronic diseases such as cancer, heart disease, and stroke by neutralizing free radicals and preventing oxidative stress.

In a study conducted on human cells, Lion's Mane Mushroom extract was found to have significant antioxidant properties, reducing oxidative stress and protecting cells from damage. Another study found that the polysaccharides present in this mushroom were able to protect cells from oxidative stress, suggesting a potential role for Lion's Mane Mushroom in reducing the risk of chronic diseases.

Neuroprotective Properties

One of the most well-known medicinal properties of Lion's Mane Mushroom is its neuroprotective properties, which make it a potential natural remedy for neurological disorders such as Alzheimer's disease and Parkinson's disease. Compounds present in this mushroom, such as hericystin and erinacine, have been shown to have neuroprotective effects by promoting nerve growth and function.

In one study, mice fed a diet supplemented with Lion's Mane Mushroom extract showed improved cognitive function and increased nerve growth factor (NGF) production. This protein is essential for the growth and survival of neurons. Another human study found that consuming Lion's Mane Mushroom extract daily for 16 weeks significantly improved mild cognitive impairment. This condition often precedes the development of dementia and Alzheimer's disease.

Cardiovascular Health

Lion's Mane Mushroom may also positively impact cardiovascular health by reducing the risk of heart disease. This mushroom contains compounds such as beta-glucans and eritadenine, which have been shown to have cholesterol-lowering properties and improve blood circulation.

A study in rats found that supplementing the diet with Lion's Mane Mushroom extract significantly reduced blood cholesterol levels and improved blood circulation. Another human study found that consuming Lion's Mane Mushroom extract daily for four weeks decreased systolic blood pressure, indicating a potential role for this mushroom in reducing the risk of heart disease.

Anticancer Properties

Lion's Mane Mushroom has also been found to have potential anticancer properties, making it a promising natural remedy for various types of cancer. Compounds present in this mushroom, such as polysaccharides and beta-glucans, have been shown to have antiproliferative and pro-apoptotic effects, which can help reduce the growth and spread of cancer cells.

In a study conducted on human cancer cells, Lion's Mane Mushroom extract was found to have antiproliferative effects, reducing the growth of cancer cells. Another study found that the polysaccharides present in this mushroom could induce apoptosis (cell death) in human cancer cells, suggesting a potential role for Lion's Mane Mushroom in reducing cancer risk.

In conclusion, Lion's Mane Mushroom is a highly valued edible fungus used for medicinal purposes for centuries in traditional Chinese and Japanese medicine. Over the years, numerous scientific studies have confirmed the therapeutic properties of this mushroom, making it a promising natural remedy for various health conditions, including neurological disorders, inflammation, cardiovascular disease, and cancer. The compounds in Lion's Mane Mushroom, such as hericystin, erinacine, beta-glucans, and polysaccharides, have been shown to have various hericystin, erinacine, beta-glucans, and polysaccharides have a variety of therapeutic effects, including neuroprotective effects, anti-inflammatory effects, cholesterol-lowering properties, and anticancer effects. Although more research is needed to fully understand the medicinal properties of Lion's Mane Mushroom, the available evidence suggests that it has the potential to be a valuable natural remedy for various health conditions.

Check out the best lion's mane mushroom supplement!

6

Cordyceps Mushroom Medicinal Properties and Health Benefits

One of the medicinal mushrooms, Cordyceps Sinensis, is rich in cordycepin, a chemical component. There is evidence that this chemical can increase athletic performance and treat respiratory infections.

Recently, cordyceps popularity has risen as a result of its capacity to replicate the effects of exercise on blood vessels. Also known as the caterpillar fungus, cordyceps is a mushroom species with a long, finger-like body hence their nickname.

Affected hosts have long, thin branches sprouting from their bodies when these fungi infect them. Due to its various health benefits, Cordyceps extract supplements and products have grown increasingly popular.

More than 400 species of Cordyceps were found, but only two have been studied in depth for their potential health benefits: Cordyceps militaris and Cordyceps Sinensis.

The body must produce the chemical adenosine triphosphate (ATP) to supply muscles with the energy they need. Cordyceps are thought to boost this production. This can enhance your body's ability to utilize oxygen, particularly when exercising.

Participants who took CS-4 had their VO2 max rise by 7%, whereas those who took a dummy pill saw no change. VO2 max is an indicator of a person's level of physical fitness.

Due to cordyceps beta-glucan content, it has anti-inflammatory qualities. A small amount of inflammation in the body is beneficial. Still, it can also lead to many undesirable outcomes, such as heart and blood vessel disease, diabetes, cancer, and autoimmune illnesses like rheumatism.

Many autoimmune diseases could benefit from the mushroom's anti-inflammatory properties, as evidenced by studies showing that exposure to Cordyceps reduces the body's production of pro-inflammatory proteins.

Cordycepin, a naturally occurring compound in cordyceps, was studied in rats in an Asian study to determine if it could help them get more restful sleep. According to a survey, cordycepin has increased non-rapid eye movement sleep in rats. Cordycepin may be beneficial to sleep-disturbed patients as a result of this experiment.

Cordyceps mushroom medicinal properties

Cordyceps' d-mannitol cordycepin and 3'-deoxyadenosine, two of its active ingredients, regulate insulin and blood sugar levels. In animal models, Cordyceps supplements have been shown to lower blood sugar and insulin levels.

Athletics performance

According to some research, the fungus can stimulate the body's production of the energy-carrying molecule ATP. Blood is pumped more efficiently to ensure that more oxygen and ATP are delivered to the organs and cells throughout the body due to higher ATP generation. Unlike other stimulants like coffee and guarana, this supplement doesn't have the unpleasant side effects that come with them.

The possibility that cordyceps can decrease tumor growth has recently sparked curiosity. Human cancer cells from the lungs, colon, skin, and liver have all been found to be inhibited in test tubes by Cordyceps.

Digestive and absorption processes are among the most well-known, but many others exist. Diet and supplementation can ensure that the liver receives all the nutrients and cofactors

it needs to function optimally. Cordyceps Sinensis's excellent list of functions includes hepatoprotective effects, which should be no surprise. This study demonstrated that mitochondrial support and the

inhibition of liver cell death helped protect the liver from injury.

The kidneys filter about 180 liters daily, which is a significant amount of blood for cleansing and disposal. The best method to ensure your kidneys' long-term health with such a demanding workload is to provide them with as much assistance as possible.

Cordyceps Sinensis can improve kidney and immunological function for patients with renal failure while reducing the amount of anti-rejection medication needed following a kidney transplant. Renal fibrosis treatment and prevention is another area where it shows potential.

Chinese diabetics have long utilized Cordyceps, but this field's scientific study is limited. Cordyceps pills for four weeks reduced weight and lowered cholesterol in diabetic rats, according to a 2012 study.

The researchers found no evidence that the supplements

influenced blood sugar levels or improved insulin resistance, but they did observe that weight loss may be significant in managing diabetes.

Check out the best Cordyceps Medicinal Mushroom Supplement!

7

Tremella Mushroom Health Benefits and Medicinal Properties

The Tremella mushroom, also known as Snow Fungus, Silver Ear Fungus, or Yun-er in Chinese, has been an edible fungus in traditional Chinese medicine for centuries. In recent years, there has been growing interest in its potential health benefits and scientific research into the various compounds in this mushroom. This chapter will delve into the multiple health benefits and medicinal properties of the Tremella mushroom and explore the scientific evidence behind these claims.

Antioxidant Properties

One of the most well-known health benefits of the Tremella mushroom is its potent antioxidant properties. Antioxidants help to protect the body from damage caused by free radicals, which are unstable molecules that can cause cellular damage leading to several health problems, including heart disease, cancer, and age-related diseases. The Tremella mushroom is rich in compounds such as polysaccharides, flavonoids, and superoxide dismutase (SOD), all of which have been shown to have strong antioxidant properties.

19

A study conducted in 2009 found that the polysaccharides extracted from the Tremella mushroom had vigorous antioxidant activity and the ability to scavenge free radicals and prevent lipid peroxidation. Another study found that the SOD activity of the Tremella mushroom was comparable to that of other medicinal mushrooms, such as the Reishi mushroom and the Agaricus blazei mushroom.

Anti-Aging Properties

In addition to its antioxidant properties, the Tremella mushroom is also believed to have anti-aging properties. The compounds found in the Tremella mushroom, such as polysaccharides, flavonoids, and SOD, have been shown to have anti-inflammatory and anti-aging effects on the skin. This is because they help protect the skin from damage caused by free radicals and promote collagen production, which is essential for maintaining skin elasticity and firmness.

A study conducted in 2016 found that topical application of Tremella mushroom extract significantly improved skin hydration, elasticity, and roughness in women aged 40-60. Another study found that Tremella mushroom extract stimulated the production of hyaluronic acid, a key component of skin hydration and youthfulness.

Immune System Boost

The Tremella mushroom is also believed to have immune-boosting properties. The polysaccharides found in the mushroom have been shown to have potent immunomodulatory effects, which means they can help to regulate and enhance the immune system. This can help protect the body from various health problems, including infections, chronic diseases, and cancer.

A study conducted in 2015 found that supplementing with

Tremella mushroom extract significantly increased the production of cytokines, which are critical mediators of the immune system, in healthy individuals. Another study found that Tremella mushroom extract was able to enhance the immune response to a flu vaccine, indicating that it may have potential as an adjuvant for immunization.

Anti-Tumor Properties

The Tremella mushroom is also believed to have anti-tumor properties. The polysaccharides found in the mushroom have been shown to have potent anti-tumor effects and to be able to inhibit the growth and spread of cancer cells. This is thought to be due to the ability of the polysaccharides to stimulate the immune system and directly inhibit the growth and spread of cancer cells.

A study conducted in 2015 found that supplementing with Tremella mushroom extract significantly reduced the size and number of tumors in mice with breast cancer.

Check out the best Tremella Medicinal Mushroom Supplement!

8

Reishi Mushrooms Medicinal Properties and Health Benefits

A single serving of reishi mushrooms contains more than 400 unique nutrients. Triterpenoids, a class of chemicals linked to a reduced risk of diabetes and heart disease, are included in this category. According to studies, consuming mushrooms can shield the body against cell deterioration, which can cause many chronic diseases.

The growth of tumors can be slowed or stopped by a substance called beta-glucan in reishi mushrooms.

In laboratory testing, reishi mushroom extracts have increased natural killer cells, a subset of white blood cells that go after abnormal and cancerous cells. One suffers from chronic fatigue if obtaining enough sleep does not make one feel less worn out. According to experts, long-term exhaustion may result from various factors, including infections, immune system diseases, hormonal imbalances, and stress. Researchers believe reishi mushrooms can lessen the symptoms of chronic fatigue syndrome (CFS).

22

Reishi Mushrooms' immune-boosting and free radical-fighting properties may account for this impact. Reishi mushrooms can positively affect testosterone levels so that you can maintain high energy levels. Because white blood cells fight viruses, germs, and other diseases as they travel through the body, the reishi mushroom's promise to improve long-term health may be true. White blood cell production and function

may be improved by consuming reishi mushrooms, according to research.

As a traditional cancer treatment, the reishi mushroom has a long history of use, and plenty of scientific data supports its claims. Reishi mushrooms can help with breast and prostate cancer. These polysaccharides, notably Beta-D-glucans, and triterpenes, have shown significant anti-inflammatory and cytotoxic effects against cancer cell lines and the ability to suppress tumor growth.

The most fascinating and maybe the most significant health advantage of Reishi is its ability to reduce stress and anxiety. Reishi is a valuable ally in our fast-paced and excessively stressed environment because of this. Chronic stress is one of the primary factors in the development of disease. Reishi is used in Traditional Chinese Medicine (TCM) to improve Chi, or Qi, the source of our life force energy, and boost metabolic activity. Chi tonics, in contrast, don't have stimulants.

Reishi has numerous health advantages for CFS patients. These health benefits include balancing and supporting critical bodily systems like the immune system, the heart, the liver, and the kidneys; reducing inflammation; increasing oxygen utilization; and supporting detoxification.

Cardiovascular disease is a prominent cause of death in developing countries. Several studies have shown that Reishi is a good source of nutrients for the heart. Many studies have shown that taking Reishi can improve cardiovascular health because of its high antioxidants. The three types of antioxidants are flavonoids, polysaccharides, and sterols. These antioxidants can reduce many risk factors for heart disease and stroke.

The liver, the second-largest organ in the body, has a variety of cleansing and digestion functions. Environmental contaminants, junk food consumption, emotional stress, and other unhealthy lifestyle choices affect the liver. By reducing the toxic load on our livers, we can better methylate, detoxify, and repair our bodies. Our bodies operate more effectively and efficiently when our livers are in good condition. Reishi mushrooms are an excellent way to enhance the function of the liver.

Check out the best Reishi Medicinal Mushroom Supplements!

9

Turkey Tail Mushroom Medicinal Properties and Health Benefits

Turkey tail mushrooms are high in fiber and low in calories. The medicinal benefits of turkey tail mushrooms can help everything from the immune system to losing weight!

The only mushrooms that contain vitamin D, proven to enhance mood, sleep patterns, and bone health, are turkey tails. Niacin, potassium, folate, selenium, riboflavin, copper, phosphorus, and B vitamins are also abundant.

Turkey tail mushrooms are also good for the immune system due to their high vitamin content. Researchers have found that turkey tail mushrooms can protect against some types of cancer, including breast cancer, thanks to their beta-glucans. Beta-glucans are a type of fiber that have uses in immunotherapy.

Turkey tail mushrooms are a good source of fiber and help with digestion. These properties are essential for proper gut function and relieve the body of toxic substances stored in the colon. These benefits help keep your immune system strong and reduce your risk of diabetes and cancer.

Turkey tail mushrooms offer powerful liver benefits. The fiber in turkey tail mushrooms helps cleanse your liver and regulate your blood sugar. One of the most potent antioxidants found in turkey tail mushrooms, selenium, also helps prevent and reduce inflammation of the liver and digestive system.

Turkey tail mushrooms are a great source of organic antibiotics. The growth of germs in tonsillitis, pharyngitis, sinusitis and bronchitis are positively affected when supplementing turkey tail mushrooms. People with arthritis or other chronic pain can also benefit from the anti-inflammatory properties of turkey tail mushrooms.

Turkey tail mushrooms inhibit histamine release, which minimizes contact inflammation. People with chronic pain have reported significantly less pain after briefly swallowing turkey tail mushrooms.

Check out the best Turkey Tail Medicinal Mushroom Supplement!

10

Maitake Mushroom Medicinal Properties and Health Benefits

The edible fungus known as the maitake mushroom in Japan is officially called by the scientific name Grifola frondosa. This culinary and medicinal fungus has strengthened the immune system and lengthened one's lifespan.

The bioactive polysaccharides D-fraction, MD-fraction, and SX-fraction, are particularly abundant in maitake mushroom extracts. Numerous studies have shown protein polysaccharides to protect the immune system and fight tumors.

Supports immune system

Beta-glucan has the potential to assist in boosting one's immune system function. It has a powerful effect on the immune system because of the D-fraction in maitake mushrooms. It improves one's immune response by increasing the synthesis of lymphokines, protein mediators, and interleukins, released proteins. SX-fraction, another beta-glucan, has been demonstrated to reduce blood glucose levels in clinical testing. Diabetic treatment is made more accessible with the help of this supplement.

Certain mushroom types have more significant levels of ergosterol, the vitamin D-producing molecule, than others. As they are harvested from the wild, maitake mushrooms' natural vitamin D concentration rises with exposure to sunlight. Typically, mushrooms contain between 28 micrograms to 1123 IU of vitamin D. This is almost 200% of the recommended daily allowance for this vitamin. Calcium absorption, which is crucial for strong bones, is aided by vitamin D.

To lessen the risk of heart disease, beta-glucan in maitake can help lower one's cholesterol and improve cardiovascular health and arterial function. Polysaccharides can reduce LDL (bad) cholesterol found in maitake, which does not affect triglyceride or HDL (good) cholesterol levels.

The potential for beta-glucan as a cancer treatment is very promising. Several investigations have demonstrated it to be beneficial against various malignant tumors. Other studies have shown that adding vitamin C to the D- and MD-fractions can help cancer therapy.

Senescence is mainly brought on by neurodegenerative changes, diminished antioxidant enzyme activity, and insufficient immune responses, including low body weight, hair loss, sluggish conduct, and laziness. MT-glucan, a substance found in maitake mushrooms, delays senescence and boosts antioxidation or immunomodulation, acting as an anti-aging agent.

Maitake medicinal properties

Respiratory disorders can benefit from maitake mushrooms' anti-inflammatory and antiviral effects. Supplements containing maitake mushrooms boost the immune system's ability to combat various diseases, alleviate symptoms, and shorten their duration. The antibacterial capabilities of acetic and malic acids are present in maitake and can be used to kill microorganisms. Maitake can also treat conditions like sinusitis and bronchitis.

Experimental evidence suggests that the immune system benefits from maitake D-fraction. Maitake mushrooms have not been proven to help treat or prevent cancer in humans by peer-reviewed medical publications; however, several human studies are now underway. Promoters of maitake mushroom extract believe it stimulates the immune system and reduces or reverses tumor growth. According to research, maitake mushrooms can help reduce the harmful effects of chemotherapy, such as nausea and hair loss.

In the therapy of the immunodeficiency virus, its capacity to stimulate the immune system could be attractive. The combination of maitake can help prevent many diseases that prey on the immune system's vulnerability due to AIDs.

In treating circulatory system disorders, the Maitake mushroom's anti-bloating, antihypertensive, and anticholesterol qualities make it a good treatment option. Blood-thinning and preventing clot formation are benefits of lowering blood pressure and cholesterol regulation for preventing heart attacks and other artery-clogging conditions.

People with diabetes can benefit as it helps regulate blood sugar since it increases glucose levels when they are low and reduces them when they are high.

PCOS is the most common endocrine illness in women of reproductive age, and it can cause various issues, including irregular menstruation, hyperandrogenism, and metabolic problems. Women with PCOS can take water-soluble glyco-protein as a monotherapy to help them get their period back on track.

Check out the best Maitake Medicinal Mushroom Supplement!

11

Chaga Mushroom Medicinal Properties and Health Benefits

One fungus showing promising therapeutic benefits is the Inonotus Obliquus, commonly known as the Chaga mushroom. Chaga mushrooms contain vital medicinal and active substances that can aid in the prevention and treatment of cancer.

This mushroom also contains anti-inflammatory and antimicrobial properties that help you fight off disease-causing microbes and prevent you from getting diseases associated with long-term inflammation.

When consumed routinely, Chaga aids in the reduction of blood sugar and cholesterol levels.

What are the medicinal properties of the Chaga mushroom?

The Chaga mushrooms contain the following medicinal properties/compounds; Antioxidants, Betulin, Betulinic acid, lignins, Melanins, Notablyinotodiol, Polysaccharides, and Triterpenoids.

Chaga mushrooms are a powerful superfood that can provide many health benefits. They are rich in vitamins, minerals, and antioxidants, which may help prevent chronic diseases like heart disease and cancer. Chaga mushrooms may also boost the immune system by encouraging the production of white blood cells that fight infections. Immune system health is also increased by compounds called beta-glucans found in these mushrooms.

Chaga mushrooms are rich in vitamins, minerals, antioxidants, flavonoids, enzymes, and dietary fiber. Chaga mushrooms contain more vitamin C than oranges (390mg vs. 60mg). If you're looking for a natural way to boost your immune system or improve your overall health this winter season, look no further than Chaga tea!

Chaga is exceptionally hardy and can even survive being frozen just below the surface of the water for months at a time - making it one of the most resilient mushrooms we know about today. Chaga mushrooms contain compounds that have anti-inflammatory properties. These anti-inflammatory compounds can help reduce inflammation in the body and may help with arthritis, digestive problems, and other inflammatory conditions. Chaga mushrooms are also rich in antioxidants.

Chaga mushrooms may help boost the immune system by encouraging the production of white blood cells that fight infections. Immune system health is also increased by compounds called beta-glucans found in these mushrooms.

Chaga mushrooms are rich in beta-glucans, classified as polysaccharides that have been shown to stimulate the immune system. These compounds can help fight infections and reduce inflammation, making them a great addition to any supplement regimen. Chaga mushrooms may help boost the immune system by encouraging the production of white blood cells that fight infections. Immune system health is also increased by compounds called beta-glucans found in these mushrooms.

Free radicals are known to cause oxidative damage to cells in the body and contribute to several chronic diseases, such as cancer and heart disease. Antioxidants can neutralize these free radicals, promoting overall health and preventing disease.

In addition to being a rich source of antioxidant compounds, Chaga mushrooms also contain other compounds that are shown to have anti-inflammatory effects. These include phenolic acids like salicylic acid, quinones like anthraquinone C1, and triterpenes (a plant molecule) like betulinic acid, botulinal acetate, and piceonolide I.

Various health benefits could be obtained from Chaga mushrooms because of their unique combination of nutrients and chemicals. Chaga mushrooms have been used for centuries in Chinese and European folk medicine. They can be applied topically to heal wounds, ingested to help with stomach ulcers, digestive problems, and intestinal worms, taken as a tea for diabetes treatment and prevention, or used in tinctures and salves to treat cancer. Chaga has also been researched for its anti-inflammatory properties that could help people with arthritis or Crohn's disease; however, these claims have not yet been proven scientifically.

Overall, Chaga mushrooms may be an excellent addition to your diet. They are rich in vitamins, minerals, antioxidants, flavonoids, and enzymes. Chaga mushrooms contain potent anti-inflammatory properties that can help reduce inflammatory symptoms such as arthritis and digestive problems. Chaga mushroom may also boost immune system health by encouraging the production of white blood cells that fight infections or cancer cells!

Check out the best Chaga Mushroom Supplement!

12

Oyster Mushroom Medicinal Properties and Health Benefits

Oyster mushrooms are a type of edible fungi that have many different health benefits. They are a good source of vitamins and minerals and contain compounds that can help boost the immune system, fight cancer cells, and improve heart health.

One of oyster mushrooms' most well-known health benefits is their ability to fight cancer cells. Polysaccharides and other compounds in oyster mushrooms can help stimulate the immune system and destroy cancer cells. Studies have shown that oyster mushroom extract can help slow the growth of liver, breast, and colon cancer cells.

Another one of the health benefits of oyster mushrooms is their ability to improve heart health. Oyster mushrooms include substances like lovastatin and eritadenine that can help decrease cholesterol levels and enhance blood vessel function. Additionally, antioxidants like selenium and copper, which can help prevent heart disease, are abundant in oyster mushrooms.

As mentioned earlier, oyster mushrooms contain compounds like polysaccharides that can help stimulate the immune system.

Studies have shown that these compounds can help increase the production of white blood cells responsible for fighting off infection. Polysaccharides can also help increase the production of antibodies, which can further protect against disease.

Oyster mushrooms are a type of edible fungi with many different medicinal properties. They're a good source of vitamins and minerals and contain compounds that can help boost the immune system, fight cancer cells, and improve heart health. If you're looking for an easy way to add more nutrition to your diet, consider incorporating some recipes with oyster mushrooms into your meal plan or supplementing them with a capsule.

Check out the best Oyster Mushroom Supplement!

13

Agarikon Mushroom Medicinal Properties and Health Benefits

There are many medicinal mushrooms, but Agarikon is one of the select few that can treat various ailments. As well as Quinine Conk and The Bread of Ghosts, other common names for the Agarikon fungus include Tree Biscuit, LaricifomesLaricifomes Officinalis, and Fomitopsis.

Bioactive chemicals found in mushrooms have been used to treat everything from cancer to infections to addiction and depression. An excellent example of this is the Agarikon mushroom. In addition to providing immunological support, it includes polyphenols, polysaccharides, carotene, and indole compounds that have several health benefits.

The Agarikon mushroom's antibacterial properties make it a valuable tool in the fight against infection. This fungus is thought by specialists to be effective in treating numerous ailments due to numerous unknown chemicals. E. coli and candida infections can be successfully treated using Agarikon mushrooms.

Supplementing with Agarikon mushrooms can positively

affect the immune system, assisting in preventing disease. Agarikon mushrooms contain immune-boosting polysaccharides such as beta-D glucan and other polysaccharides. In addition, Agarikon mushrooms aid in pain relief and the reduction of arthritic, lumbago, and other medical conditions.

The immunotherapeutic effects of the Agarikon mushroom are well-known. Immunomodulatory features of the mushroom, such as activating dendritic cells, macrophages, T-cells, cytokines, and NK cells, have traditionally been utilized to support the immune system. Antibiotics, viruses, poisons, and even allergens can all be conquered with a robust immune system.

The beneficial effects of Agarikon mushrooms include their anti-proliferative capabilities. Like the anticancer 5-fluorouracil, it has shown anti-proliferative abilities against cancer cells. Studies show that agarikon mushrooms have anti-proliferative properties in HeLa cervical cancer and colon cancer.

Beneficial properties of Agarikon mushrooms include respiratory assistance. People around the globe are affected by respiratory disorders. Due to their ubiquity, there has been a massive investment in the fight against respiratory diseases to help patients manage their conditions and improve their general health.

If not treated promptly, tuberculosis can be lethal. Mycobacterium tuberculosis is the bacteria that causes tuberculosis. The chlorinated coumarins found in Agarikon mushrooms are useful against tuberculosis. A further active ingredient in the mushroom is agaric acid. This acid is known to have antibacterial, parasympatholytic, and anhidrotic effects.

The anti-inflammatory qualities of the Agarikon mushroom

make it an effective treatment for arthritis pain and inflammation. Swollen joints are a common symptom of arthritis, which may wreak havoc on the body. L-ergothioneine, a potent antioxidant, is found in high concentrations in this mushroom, which reports helping people with pain in their joints.

Kidney illness may benefit from the use of Agarikon mushrooms. Drinking Agarikon mushroom tea daily can help treat kidney infections, edema, and other issues with the urinary tract.

Smallpox killed thousands of Americans in the United States in 1947. Vaccines have been produced, but tests have shown that they are 95% effective in protecting against disease. There is evidence that the agarikon mushroom contains antiviral properties against the variola virus, which causes smallpox. These antiviral capabilities include herpes, influenza A, and B, as well as other viruses.

Check out the best Agarikon Mushroom Supplement!

<h1 style="text-align:center">14</h1>

Poria Mushroom and Cancer

A species of fungus called the poria mushroom has long been employed in traditional Chinese medicine. Poria mushrooms are white or tan and grow on tree roots. In medicine, the entire fungus is used.

The antioxidants and polysaccharides found in poria mushrooms are thought to be the source of the mushroom's health advantages. Let's examine some of the ways the Poria mushroom can enhance your health in more detail.

Cancer prevention is one of the health advantages of poria mushrooms that has received the most attention. Studies on animals and in test tubes have revealed that Poria mushrooms have the power to eradicate cancer cells and prevent their growth. It was also discovered to improve the efficiency of some cancer medications.

Poria mushroom may also help support diabetes. One study showed that it improved insulin sensitivity and lowered blood sugar levels in rats with diabetes. Another study found that it increased antioxidant levels and reduced inflammation in rats with diabetes.

Alzheimer's disease is a degenerative brain disorder that leads to memory loss and cognitive decline. Poria mushroom may help treat Alzheimer's disease by reducing inflammation and protecting brain cells from damage.

15

Can Mushrooms Help Your Hair Grow?

Some people are now utilizing mushrooms to grow their hair. Despite the lack of scientific proof, there are a few reasons why mushrooms might be able to promote hair growth.

Mushrooms are a good source of B vitamins, including niacin, riboflavin, and biotin. B vitamins are essential for healthy hair growth. Niacin helps increase blood flow to the scalp, encouraging hair growth. Riboflavin helps the body to produce new cells, including hair cells. Biotin aids in producing keratin, a key structural component of hair. Mushrooms are also a good source of copper. Copper helps to form new blood vessels, which can promote hair growth. In addition, copper helps to keep existing blood vessels open and functioning correctly.

Copper also plays a role in the production of melanin, which gives hair its color.

Mushrooms are chock-full of nutrients like selenium, copper, and zinc, which are all essential for healthy hair growth. Selenium helps to protect the scalp from damage, while copper and zinc help to strengthen the hair shaft. Mushroom extracts also contain a compound called ergothioneine, which has antioxidant and anti-inflammatory properties. All of these nutrients work together to promote healthy hair growth. But how exactly do mushrooms encourage hair growth? One theory is that mushrooms help increase blood flow to the scalp, promoting hair growth. Another idea is that mushrooms help to prevent follicle death, which can lead to hair loss. Whatever the mechanism, there's no denying that mushrooms can be effective in promoting hair growth.

If you're looking for a natural way to promote hair growth, look no further than mushrooms. Mushroom extracts are chock-full of nutrients like selenium, copper, and zinc, which are all essential for healthy hair growth. Mushroom extracts also contain a compound called ergothioneine, which has antioxidant and anti-inflammatory properties. All of these nutrients work together to promote healthy hair growth. Give mushrooms a try if you're seeking a natural solution to strengthening your hair!

16

Medicinal Mushrooms for Depression

Medicinal mushrooms have characteristics that help improve mood and cognitive function. One study found that people with depression who took a daily supplement containing mushroom extract experienced significant improvements in symptoms after eight weeks compared to those who didn't. Another study found that older adults who took a daily mushroom supplement experienced improved memory and cognitive function compared to those who didn't.

Mushrooms contain compounds that act on the body's serotonin receptors. Serotonin is a neurotransmitter crucial for controlling mood. Low serotonin levels might result in depressive and anxious feelings. Ingesting medicinal mushrooms can increase serotonin levels, enhance mood and reduce depressive symptoms.

Not all mushrooms are created equal, however. Some mushrooms, like Chaga and reishi, contain more active compounds than others. That means that they're more potent and can provide more significant benefits.

As mental health stigma dissipates, more people seek treatment for their conditions. However, traditional treatments such as medication and therapy can be ineffective or even harmful for some people. That's where psilocybin comes in. For many people suffering from depression, psilocybin therapy offers hope.

Certain kinds of mushrooms contain psilocybin, a naturally occurring hallucinogenic substance. When ingested, psilocybin produces effects similar to those of other psychedelics, such as LSD and DMT. These effects can include changes in perception, mood, and cognitive function.

Psychedelics like psilocybin work by increasing communication between different areas of the brain. This effect is thought to be mediated by the serotonin receptor 5-HT2A. In depressed individuals, there is often decreased communication between other brain regions. Psilocybin may work by increasing communication between these regions, which could help to relieve depressive symptoms.

In addition to its effects on brain function, psilocybin also leads to mystical experiences that can be therapeutic in and of themselves. These experiences can provide a sense of understanding and insight that can help deal with complex life problems. The mystical experiences induced by psychedelics are thought to be caused by changes in the Default Mode Network (DMN) activity. When we are not focused on the present moment, a network of brain areas known as the default mode network (DMN) is active because it is thought to be involved in activities like daydreaming and rumination.

The research on the effectiveness of psilocybin therapy for depression is still in its early stages. However, there have been some promising studies on the topic. One study found that psilocybin therapy was associated with decreases in self-reported measures of depression and anxiety immediately following treatment. Other studies have found similar reductions in depressive symptoms following psilocybin therapy.

The research on psilocybin therapy for depression is still in its early stages. However, the available research indicates that psilocybin may be an effective treatment for depression. Suppose you are considering trying psilocybin therapy for your depression. In that case, speaking with a qualified healthcare professional is essential to ensure that you do so safely and under proper supervision.

17

Medicinal Mushrooms for Weight Loss

There are many medicinal mushrooms, but reishi and Chaga mushrooms are the two most famous varieties for weight loss support. Both of these mushrooms are rich in antioxidants and have anti-inflammatory properties. Reishi mushrooms, in particular, offer support for boosting metabolism.

Some people believe that consuming medicinal mushrooms can help promote weight loss by aiding in fat digestion. However, there is no scientific proof to back up this assertion. Most claims about the weight loss benefits of medicinal mushrooms are based on anecdotal evidence and traditional Chinese medicine.

That being said, some preliminary research suggests that certain compounds found in medicinal mushrooms could help promote weight loss. For instance, a study in the journal Obesity discovered that mice fed a Chaga mushroom extract lost more weight than mice who did not.

While this research is promising, it's important to remember that it is still very preliminary. Whether or not medicinal mushrooms can support weight loss in people depends on further study.

18

Medicinal Mushrooms for ADHD Support

ADHD, also known as attention deficit hyperactivity disorder, is a mental illness marked by symptoms such as trouble maintaining focus, impulsive conduct, and hyperactivity. While conventional medicine relies heavily on medication to manage the symptoms of this disorder, there are other options out there that focus on natural remedies. One such remedy is medicinal mushrooms.

Lion's Mane is thought to help with cognitive function and has been shown to help repair nerve damage. A 2012 study showed that Lion's Mane helped improve attention and behavior in children with ADHD.

Turkey tail mushrooms are characterized by their multicolored appearance; they usually have stripes or swirls of brown, yellow, red, and white. These mushrooms are commonly used in Eastern medicine and have a long history of use dating back to traditional Chinese texts from the 5th century BCE. Turkey tail mushrooms are known to strengthen the immune system and have the potential to lessen ADHD symptoms. One study showed that children who took Turkey tail supplements for 16 weeks had significantly lower levels of hyperactivity than those who did not.

Reishi mushrooms are dark red or brown mushrooms that have a glossy exterior. They've been used in Traditional Chinese Medicine for centuries and are thought to be one of the most potent medicinal mushrooms. Reishi mushrooms are referred to as "adaptogens," which indicates that restoring normal bodily functions assists the body in adjusting to stimuli. Reishi mushrooms have shown promise in reducing symptoms of ADHD, particularly impulsivity and hyperactivity.

Cordyceps mushrooms are strange-looking fungi that grow on caterpillars in high-altitude regions like Tibet and Nepal. These mushrooms have been used in Traditional Chinese Medicine for hundreds of years to treat issues like fatigue and low libido. Cordyceps mushrooms are also thought to help improve cognitive function and reduce fatigue—two things that can be helpful for those with ADHD. One study showed that cordyceps supplementation improved symptoms of ADHD in children aged 6-12.

While further research is needed to confirm the efficacy of medicinal mushrooms for treating ADHD, there is some promising evidence that certain species of fungi can help improve symptoms associated with this disorder—particularly concerning impulsivity and hyperactivity.

19

Medicinal Mushrooms for Dog Health

Dogs are prone to various health issues, including cancer and joint pain. Some dog owners prefer to use natural supplements as a first line of defense, even though many other medications and therapies are available to help keep canines healthy. One such organic supplement that successfully treats various ailments in dogs is mushroom supplementation.

Reishi mushrooms have been used for millennia in traditional Chinese medicine to treat various ailments. These days, they are frequently employed as immunostimulants, supporting the immune system's stimulation. This is advantageous for dogs receiving chemotherapy or those with autoimmune diseases. Supplements containing reishi mushrooms can be effective in treating chronic pain and arthritis.

Another type of mushroom with a long history of usage in traditional medicine is the Chaga mushroom. They are beneficial in treating disorders, including arthritis and hip dysplasia, since they are used as anti-inflammatory drugs. Supplements containing chaga mushrooms can also strengthen the immune system, making them perfect for dogs prone to infections or diseases.

Although cordyceps mushrooms are a less popular supplement, they are just as effective as other varieties. Traditional uses of cordyceps mushrooms include the treatment of bronchitis and asthma. Additionally, cordyceps can treat diarrhea, tiredness, and cognitive deterioration.

Today's market offers a wide variety of supplements made from mushrooms. The advantages of each kind of mushroom supplement are different. One should consult their veterinarian before selecting a mushroom supplement for their Dog to ascertain which would work best for their unique needs.

Check out the best Medicinal Mushroom Supplement for your Dog!

20

Factors To Consider When Choosing Supplements

With so many options available, they know which one to choose can be challenging. Here are some things to consider when selecting the best medicinal mushroom supplement and what to avoid.

1. Quality of the supplement One of the most important things to consider when choosing a medicinal mushroom supplement is the quality of the product. Look for a supplement made from high-quality, organic mushrooms and free from fillers, additives, and preservatives. Additionally, ensure that the product has been tested for purity and potency and that the manufacturing process meets high standards.

2. Medicinal mushrooms have many different types, qualities, and health benefits, so choosing a supplement that contains the specific type of mushroom you're looking for is essential.

3. The extraction method used to create the supplement can

also affect its potency and quality. Look for a supplement that uses a hot water extraction method, as this is the most effective way to extract the active compounds from the mushrooms.

4. The recommended dosage of medicinal mushroom supplements can vary depending on the type of mushroom and the desired health benefits. It's essential to follow the recommended dosage and not exceed it, as taking too much can lead to adverse side effects.

5. While choosing the cheapest option available is tempting, it's important to remember that you get what you pay for. Higher-quality supplements made from high-quality, organic mushrooms and manufactured to strict standards can be more expensive. Still, they're more likely to provide the health benefits you want.

In conclusion, choosing the best medicinal mushroom supplement requires careful consideration of several vital factors. Look for a high-quality product that contains the type of mushroom you're looking for, has been manufactured using a hot water extraction method, and is free from fillers, additives, and preservatives. Remember to follow the recommended dosage and not be swayed by the cheapest option available. By taking the time to consider these factors carefully, you can ensure that you're getting the best possible supplement for your health needs.

Recommended Medicinal Mushroom Supplement Brands:

Real Mushrooms Medicinal Supplements- This brand provides high-quality mushroom supplements with no fillers and provides lab testing results of the medicinal contents.

ORIVeDA Medicinal Mushroom Supplements- Oriveda is considered one of the best mushroom supplement brands for several reasons. Firstly, the brand uses high-quality, organic mushrooms and employs a hot water extraction method to ensure maximum potency and effectiveness. Secondly, Oriveda uses a proprietary blend of multiple medicinal mushrooms, offering a more comprehensive approach to health and wellness. Thirdly, the brand strongly emphasizes quality control, conducting extensive testing to ensure its supplements are free from contaminants and meet strict purity standards. Lastly, Oriveda is dedicated to providing a sustainable and environmentally-friendly approach to mushroom cultivation, using only natural and eco-friendly methods. These factors, combined with a commitment to customer satisfaction, make Oriveda a top choice for those seeking the health benefits of medicinal mushrooms.

21

Guide to making your medicinal mushroom tinctures at home

Mushroom tinctures are concentrated forms of medicinal mushrooms that are made by soaking the mushrooms in alcohol or another solvent. Tinctures are typically taken by drops under the tongue or diluted in water. They are a good option for those who want the quickest absorption of medicinal compounds. Tinctures are also easy to take with you on the go. Some people prefer tinctures because they do not have to consume as much of the mushroom taste.

1. Start with dried mushrooms: You can use any mushroom for your tincture, but we recommend starting with dried mushrooms so they're easy to measure and weigh.

2. While glycerin will result in a sweeter, slower-acting tincture, vodka is an attractive option if you want a medicine that acts quickly and has a strong alcoholic flavor.

3. Decide on your ratio: A general ratio to follow is 1 part mushrooms to 5 parts solvent, but you can adjust this depending on your preferences.

4. Grind your mushrooms: Use a coffee grinder or blender to

grind them into a fine powder before adding them to your solvent. This will help them extract more easily. —-One can skip this step by purchasing already ground medicinal mushroom powder——

5. Add solvent and stir: Add your solvent of choice to a glass jar, then add the ground mushrooms and start well until they're thoroughly mixed in.

6. Extract for 4-6 weeks: Store your jar in a cool, dark place and allow it to extract for 4-6 weeks, shaking it once daily if possible.

7. Filter and store: After 4-6 weeks have elapsed, store your finished tincture in dark glass bottles with airtight lids by filtering away the solid residue with cheesecloth or a coffee filter. Enjoy and store in a cold, dark location.

How to make a dual extraction mushroom tincture

Mycologists have been using mushroom tinctures for years to make high-grade extracts that are potent and effective. Here is a step-by-step tutorial for performing the task yourself.

Prepare the materials.

Before you begin the process of making a dual-extraction mushroom tincture, prepare the materials you will need. When working with mushrooms, avoiding distractions and focusing solely on what you are doing is essential. Avoid watching television or checking your phone while preparing the materials. Here is a sample dual extraction recipe. Please feel free to use whichever medicinal mushrooms are best for you.

- 1/2 ounce (14 grams) dried shiitake mushrooms
- 1/2 ounce (14 grams) dried lion's mane mushrooms
- 2 cups alcohol (190 proof grain alcohol or 190 proof vodka)

Weigh and measure.

First, weigh and measure your ingredients. To do this, you'll need the following:

- Digital scales are the best option for measuring small amounts of liquid or powder.
- Measuring cup - If you don't have a digital scale, consider using a standard kitchen measuring cup to measure your ingredients instead. Using US-standard measurement units as metric (milliliters) will not work for our purposes here! You'll also need some funnel if you plan on pouring liquids into bottles; we recommend one made from glass rather than plastic because it's more durable when it comes time for storage later on down the road (after all those weeks/months/years).

Prepare the alcohol extract.

Pour the mushrooms into the glass jar. Leave about 3/4 of the pot empty.

Add enough alcohol to cover the bottom of the jar, then close it tightly and shake it vigorously for several minutes. You will see some foam form as it extracts active ingredients from your mushrooms, but don't worry about that right now—it'll settle down during filtering.

Use a coffee filter or cheesecloth to remove any leftover

mushrooms after you've reached the desired potency (usually 1-2 weeks).

Prepare the water extract.

The first step is to prepare the water extract. Add the mushrooms to a jar and then cover it with filtered water, filling the pot with about 1/3 of the total. After letting it stand for 24 hours, separate the two liquid mixtures into individual, airtight jars or containers. Put a coffee filter over another container, like a pitcher or mason jar (I like using glass ones because they look pretty), and pour your mushroom-containing solution through it slowly so as not to cause any clogging in your filter—this will help remove any particulate matter left behind from your mushrooms.

Now place both of these liquids in the freezer overnight so that they turn into ice cubes, which makes them easier to handle while adding them together later on when making tincture!

Combine extracts.

Combine extracts in a large jar. Shake to mix, then decant into smaller jars. Filter with a coffee filter or cheesecloth, and use the filtered tincture for up to one month.

Decant, filter, and bottle.

- Decant the mushroom tincture: Using a funnel, decant the mushroom tincture into a separate container.
- Filter the mushroom tincture: Allow any sediment to settle in your first container before filtering it through several

layers of cheesecloth or paper towel into another clean storage bottle (or into your original storage bottle if you want to take up less space).

- The mushroom tincture should be packaged, labeled, and kept out of sunlight and heat.

22

Powdered Medicinal Mushroom Supplements

Dried and finely ground mushrooms are used to create mushroom powders. Smoothies, coffee, tea, and other dishes can all benefit from their addition. Powders are a decent solution for individuals who don't like mushrooms' flavor or wish to cover it up with different tastes. A more effective nutrition method than whole mushrooms or tea is mushroom powder. When mushrooms are dried and ground, a larger surface area is exposed, making it more straightforward for your body to absorb the therapeutic ingredients.

To make a medicinal mushroom tea, you steep dry mushrooms in hot water to extract their beneficial compounds. Teas are a good option for those who want a less potent supplementation or want to avoid consuming alcohol or other solvents. Teas are also easy to make and can be a relaxing way to consume medicinal mushrooms. Some people enjoy the taste of mushroom teas more than tinctures or powders because steeping extracts some bitterness from the mushrooms while maintaining their flavor profile.

23

Encapsulating Medicinal Mushroom Powder

Capsules are made by encapsulating powdered mushroom extract in a plant-based casing. They are a good option for those who want an easy and convenient way to take their supplements without worrying about taste or texture. Capsules are also less potent than other methods of supplementation because only a tiny amount of powder is used per capsule.

How to Make Medicinal Mushroom Supplement Capsules

You can make your medicinal mushroom supplement capsules at home with simple ingredients and supplies. Creating one's supplement in the form of capsules is a great option to create unique blends of different mushrooms and save money simultaneously. Making your capsules ensures that you know exactly what's in them and how potent they are. Here's what you'll need:

Supplies:
  -Empty capsules #000 Size
  -Capsule Filling Machine #000 Size

-Mushroom powder (reishi, chaga, cordyceps, turkey tail, etc.)

24

Mushroom Matcha

Matcha powder, boiling water, and mushrooms are combined to create mushroom matcha. It is said to be very nourishing and to have several health advantages. Improved concentration, mental clarity, more energy, and a strengthened immune system are some of these advantages. Additionally, it is supposed to aid with weight loss. In this chapter, we'll go deeper into mushroom matcha and examine how to make it at home.

The mushrooms used in matcha tea are typically shiitake or reishi mushrooms. These mushrooms are dried and ground into powder before being added to the tea.

Add one teaspoon of mushroom powder to 1 cup of hot water to make mushroom matcha. If you want your drink to be sweeter, you can add honey or sugar to taste. You could add milk or soy milk for an even more nutritious beverage. Once all the ingredients have been added, stir well and enjoy!

Matcha with mushrooms is a tasty, healthy beverage with various advantages for your health. Give mushroom matcha a try if you're looking for an alternative to coffee or sweet drinks!

Its earthy flavor and distinctive taste will win you over. Check out this incredible Mushroom Matcha Drink!

25

Mushroom Coffee

A few years ago, brewing coffee with mushrooms might have sounded like something out of an episode of Star Trek. But today, it's a real thing, becoming increasingly popular as people learn about its unique flavor and health benefits. So what is mushroom coffee, and why should you try it?

Mushroom coffee is simply coffee brewed with mushrooms. While that might sound strange, mushrooms are a great complement to coffee. They offer a robust, earthy flavor that complements coffee beans' inherent bitterness.

Additionally, mushrooms are rich in minerals like vitamin D, potassium, and fiber, all of which have positive health effects.

There are many mushroom coffees on the market today. The two most common types are Lion's Mane mushroom coffee and Chaga mushroom coffee. Lion's Mane mushrooms are known for their cognitive-boosting properties, while Chaga mushrooms are packed with antioxidants. There are also many other mushroom coffees, each with unique flavor and health benefits.

Mushroom coffee is becoming increasingly popular due

to its unique flavor and health benefits. Some of the most notable health benefits of drinking mushroom coffee include improved cognitive function, increased energy levels, reduced inflammation, and improved digestion. Additionally, many people find that drinking mushroom coffee helps them to feel more balanced and focused throughout the day.

Brewing mushroom coffee is very similar to brewing regular drip coffee—add a scoop (or two) of ground mushrooms to your filter and your beans before brewing. You can also add mushrooms to cold brew or espresso for a unique twist on your favorite beverages. If you're feeling adventurous, try adding other ingredients like cinnamon or nutmeg to bring out the flavors of your mushrooms.

Check out this fantastic Mushroom Coffee supplement!

26

Conclusion

In conclusion, studying the health benefits and medicinal properties of medicinal mushrooms provides a comprehensive overview of various species of fungi traditionally utilized to improve health and combat multiple illnesses. Through extensive research and scientific examinations, the potent medicinal qualities of mushrooms, such as polysaccharides, beta-glucans, and terpenoids, are highlighted and found to contribute to many of the attributed health benefits.

The research delves into the myriad health benefits of medicinal mushrooms, including their ability to enhance the immune system, prevent and treat cancer, decrease inflammation, lower cholesterol levels, and improve gut health, among others. It also provides a thorough overview of the various methods of consuming medicinal mushrooms, including supplementation, teas, tinctures, and powders.

In all, the examination provides an in-depth analysis of the health benefits and medicinal properties of medicinal mushrooms, making it an essential resource for those interested in natural and alternative forms of medicine. Whether you are a healthcare professional, a natural health practitioner, or someone who seeks to promote your well-being, this study provides a wealth of information on the many health benefits of medicinal mushrooms.

The examination offers a persuasive case for using medicinal mushrooms as a safe and effective natural health supplement and highlights the incredible therapeutic potential of these fascinating fungi. Suppose you seek to explore the numerous health benefits of medicinal mushrooms. In that case, this study is a must-read that will provide you with all the information necessary to make an informed decision about incorporating these fungi into your health and wellness routine.